My Pregnancy

A Record Book

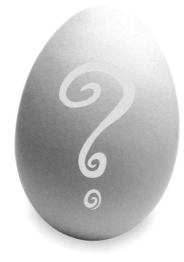

© 1997 Havoc Publishing

ISBN 1-57977-114-9

Published and created by Havoc Publishing

San Diego, California

First Printing, August 1997

Designed by Juddesign

Printed in Korea

Please write to us for more information on our

Havoc Publishing Record Books and Products.

HAVOC PUBLISHING
9808 Waples Street,
San Diego, CA 92121

My Pregnancy

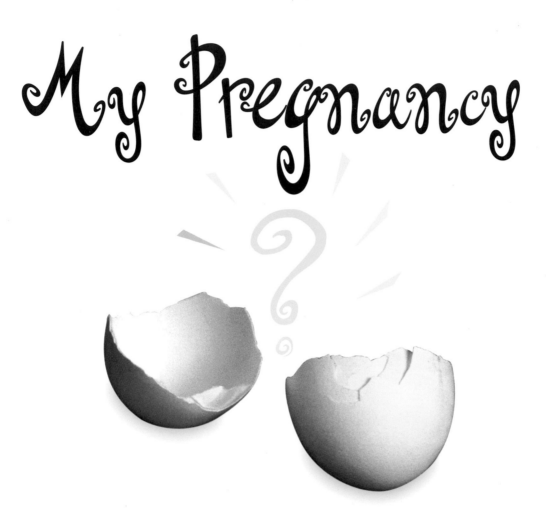

A Record Book For

Contents

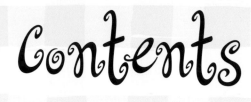

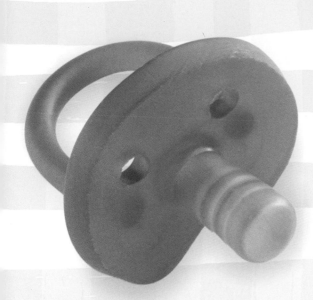

Contents

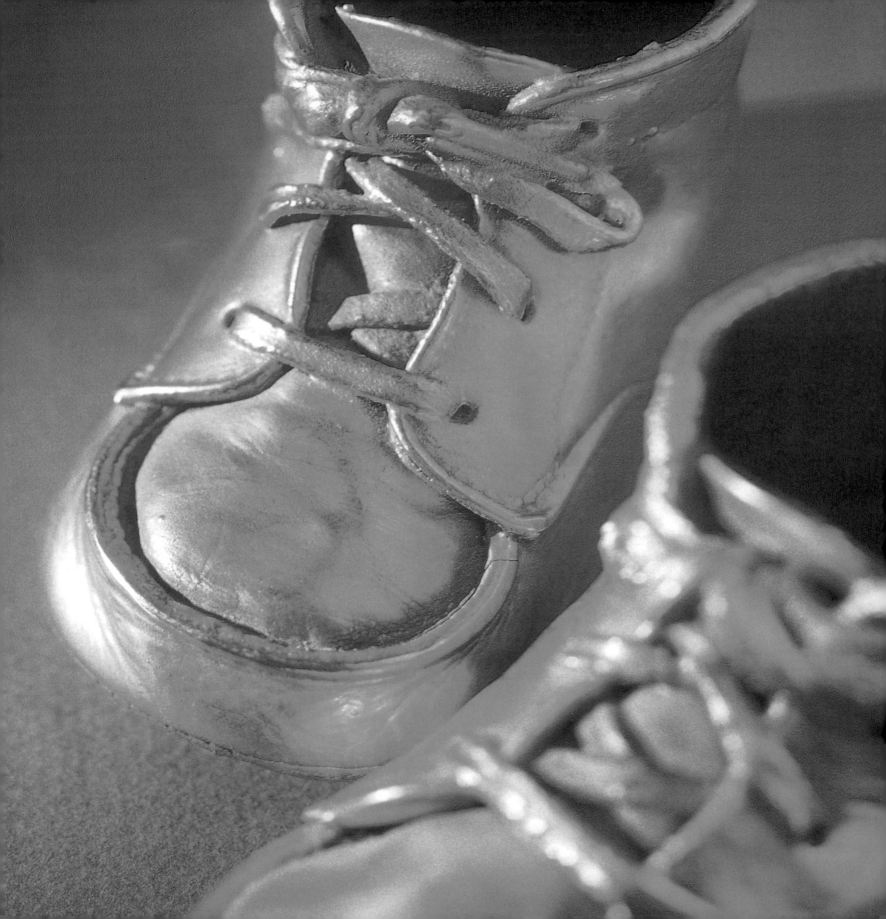

I'm Expecting!

When I suspected

Date I found out

My first doctor visit

Expected due date

My first thoughts

Celebrating the News

How we celebrated the news

_____

_____

_____

_____

Who I told first

_____

_____

Family and friends' reactions

_____

_____

_____

Anticipation

The things I am looking forward to as a mother

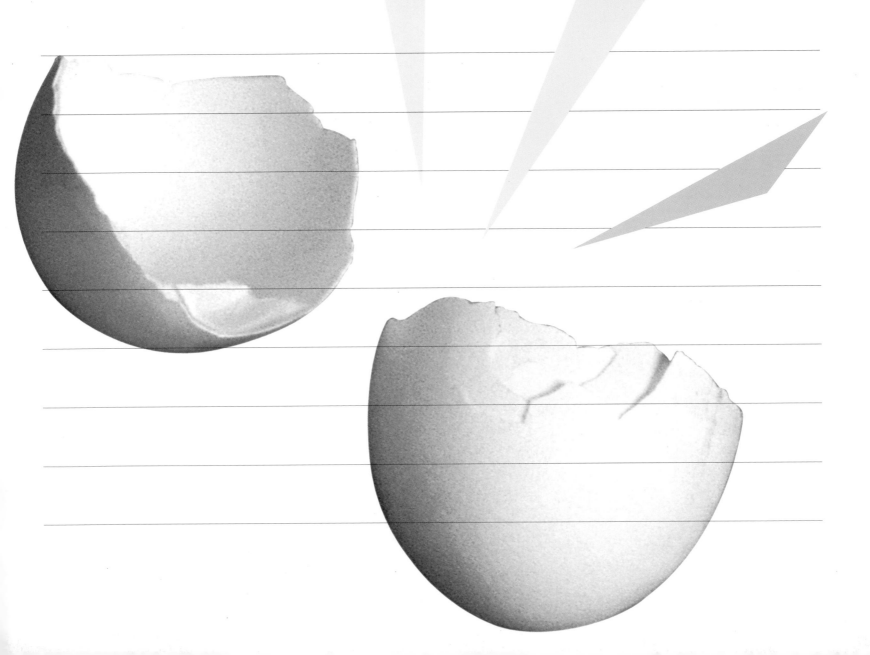

Photograph

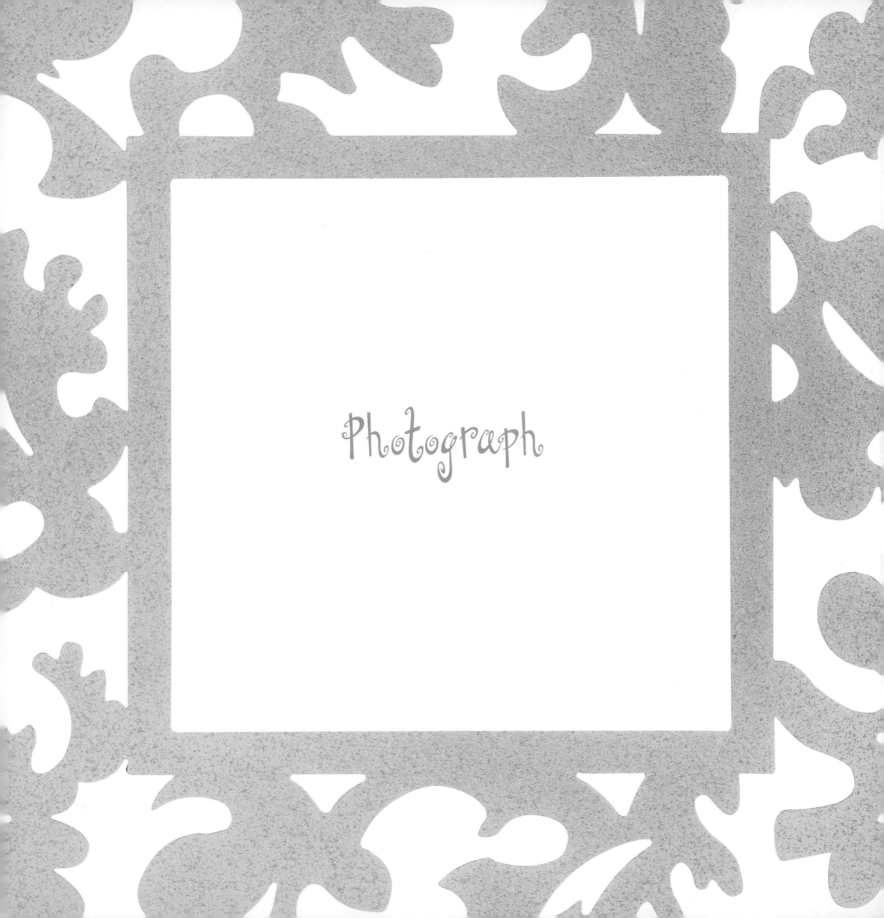

Photograph

Name

Office location

Phone number

Things to remember

Doctor's advice

eat healthy stay active take your vitamins be happy drink lots of water get plenty of rest

Goin' to the Doctor

Questions I have

_____

_____

_____

_____

_____

Important dates

_____

_____

_____

_____

_____

My Thoughts and Feelings

at 3 months

_____

_____

_____

_____

_____

_____

_____

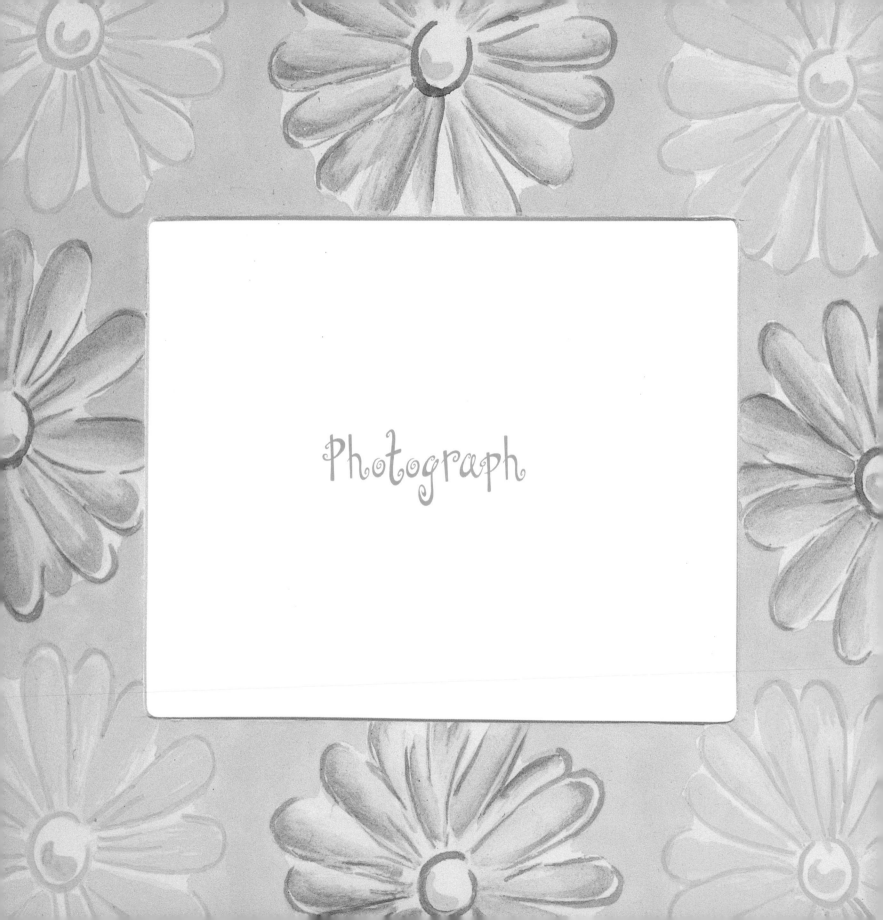

Photograph

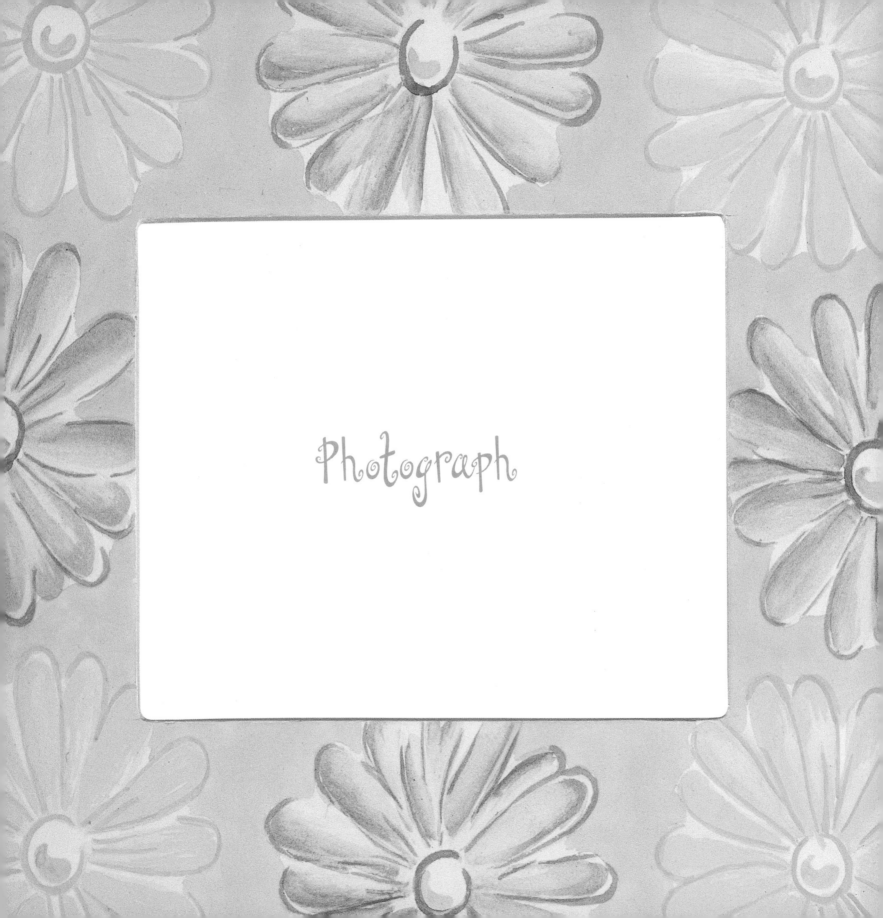

Photograph

Changing Emotions

Different emotions I've experienced along the way

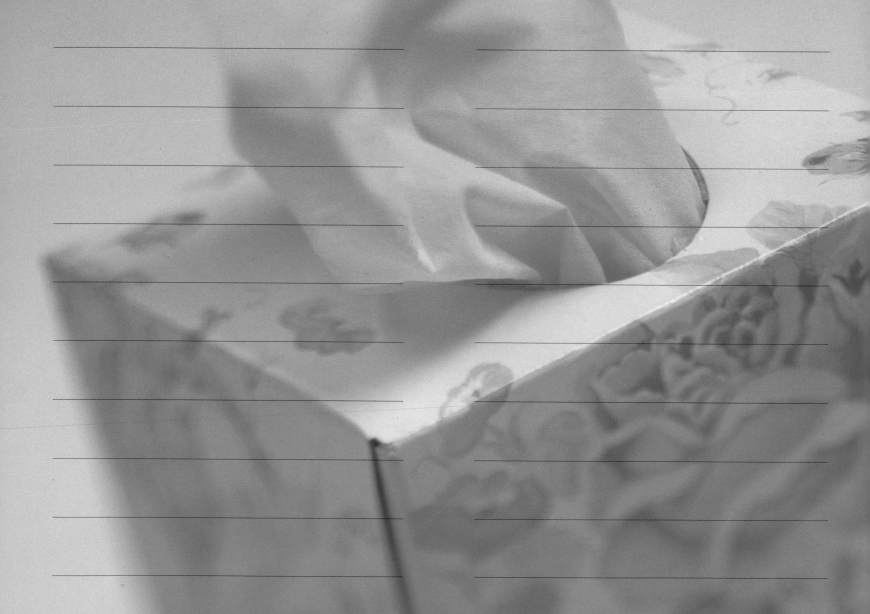

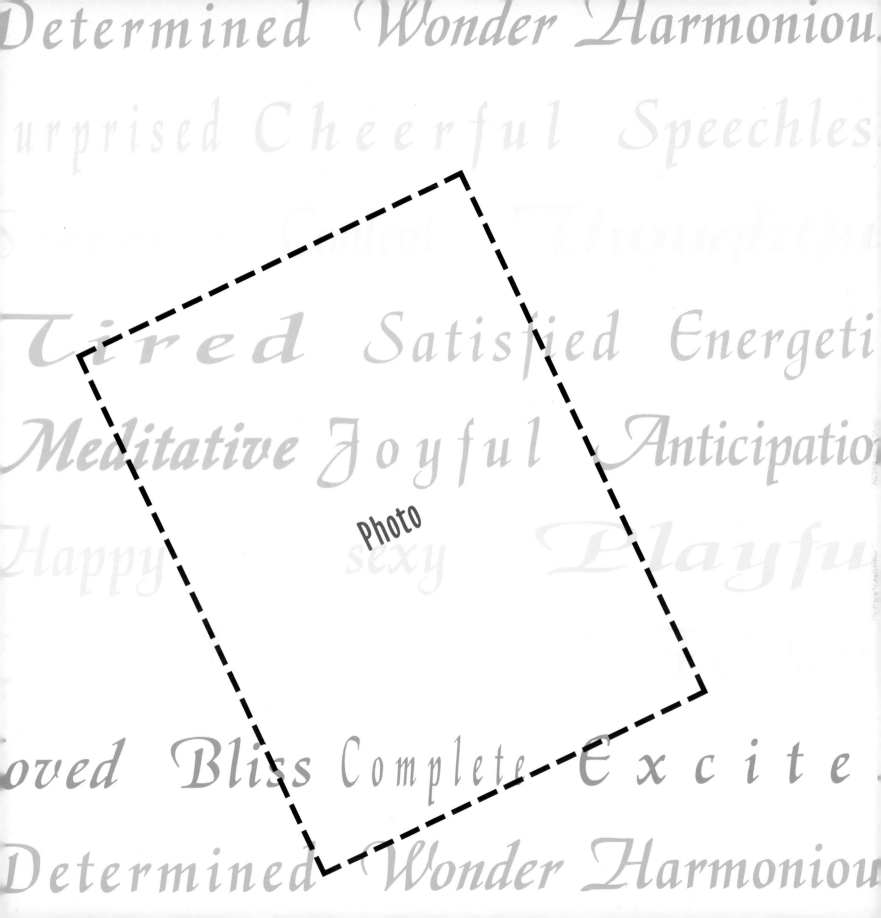

The Big Adjustments

What my pregnancy was like

Changes in lifestyle

My fashion staples

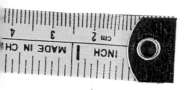

Grow...Grow...Grow

I started to really show
_____

_____

The first time you moved
_____

_____

Where you kicked most often
_____

How active were you?
_____

_____

Other physical changes and when
_____

_____

_____

Seeing you for the first time

Place ultrasound photo here

More Doctor Appointments

Date
_____

Comments
_____

Date
_____

Comments
_____

Date
_____

Comments
_____

Date
_____

Comments
_____

strange combinations

Favorite foods
_____
_____
_____
_____
_____
_____
_____
_____

Foods I craved
_____
_____
_____
_____
_____
_____

A Growing

munchies

new taste sensations

Appetite

I can't believe I ate...

_____

_____

_____

I can't believe I ate the whole thing

_____

_____

_____

Foods I just couldn't eat

_____

_____

_____

_____

fruits and vegetables

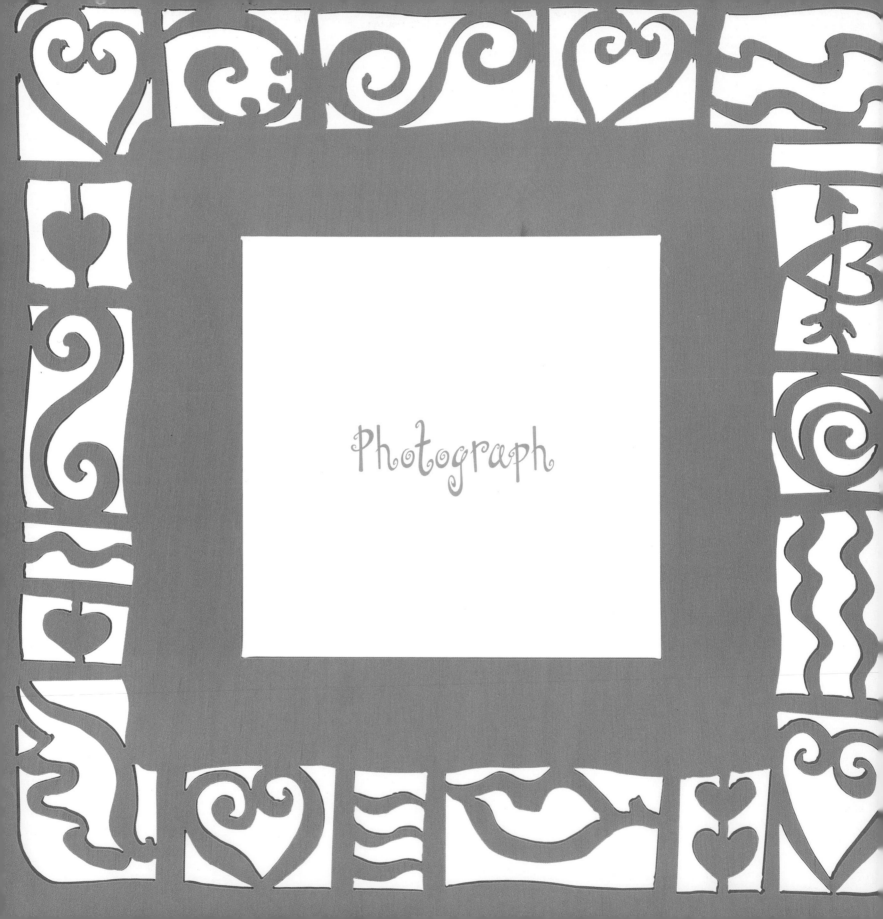

Photograph

Photograph

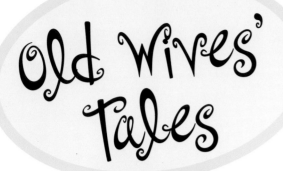

Old Wives' Tales

Do you pass the test?

Sleeping more than before?
○ It's a girl

Not so sleepy?
○ It's a boy

Is maternal Grandma's hair grey?
○ It's a boy

Is it another color?
○ It's a girl

Carrying high?
○ It's a girl

Carrying low?
○ It's a boy

Difficulty breathing?
○ It's a boy

Breathing free and easy?
○ It's a girl

Sleeping on your left side?
○ It's a boy

Sleeping on your right side?
○ It's a girl

Dreaming about having a boy?
○ It's a boy

Dreaming about having a girl?
○ It's a girl

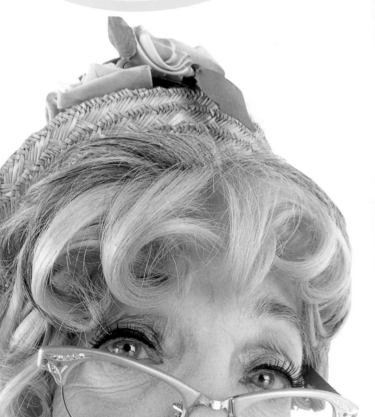

Tally up: # of boys ___

# of girls ___

Pearls Of Wisdom

Advice and shared experiences from family and friends

Are You a Boy or a Girl?

What family and friends thought you would be....

Who thinks it will be
A boy?

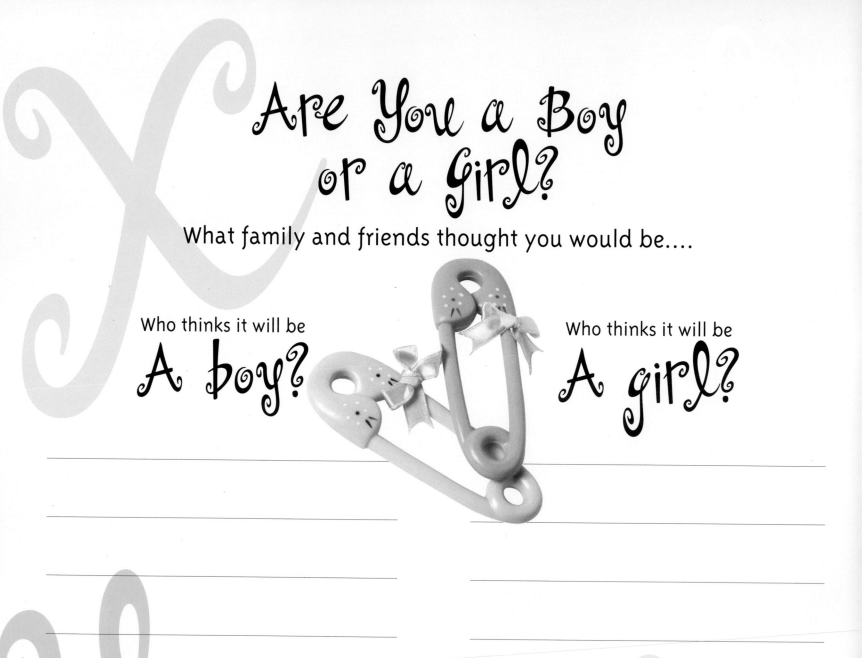

Who thinks it will be
A girl?

Guessing the Birth Date

Who	Date	Sex and weight

Treating Myself

Favorite places to relax
_____

_____

_____

_____

Music I enjoy listening to
_____

_____

_____

Activities I enjoy
_____

_____

_____

How I unwind
_____

_____

_____

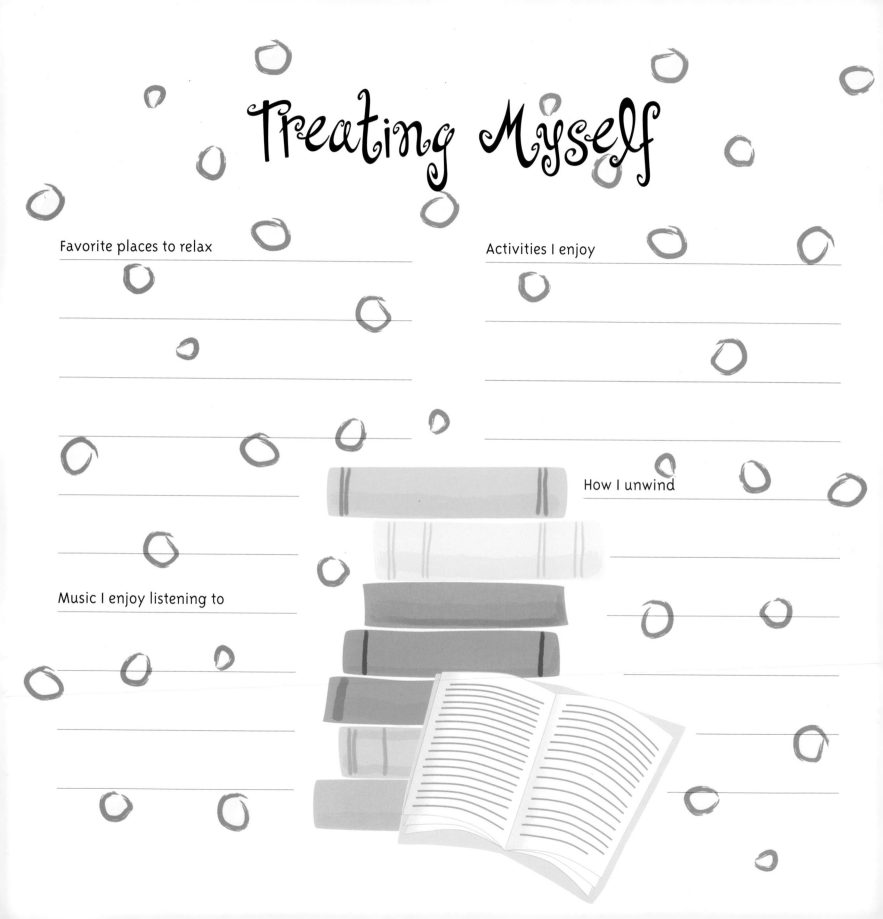

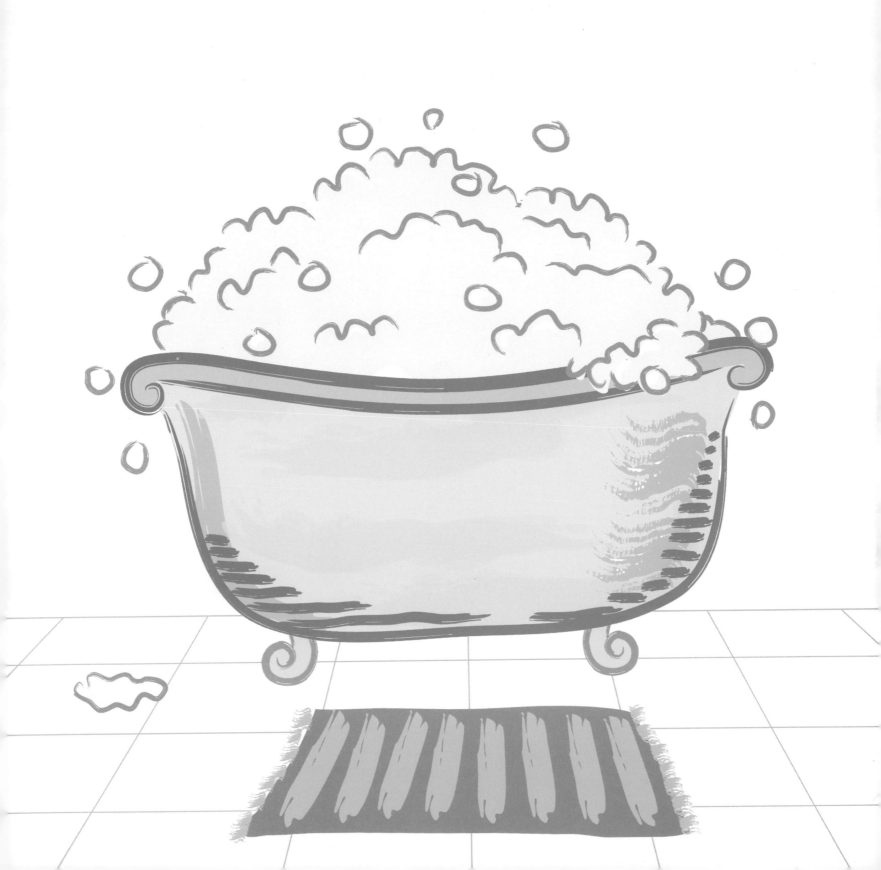

Designing the Nursery

Furnishings

_____

_____

Color scheme

_____

_____

_____

Accessories

_____

_____

_____

The Plans

Photo

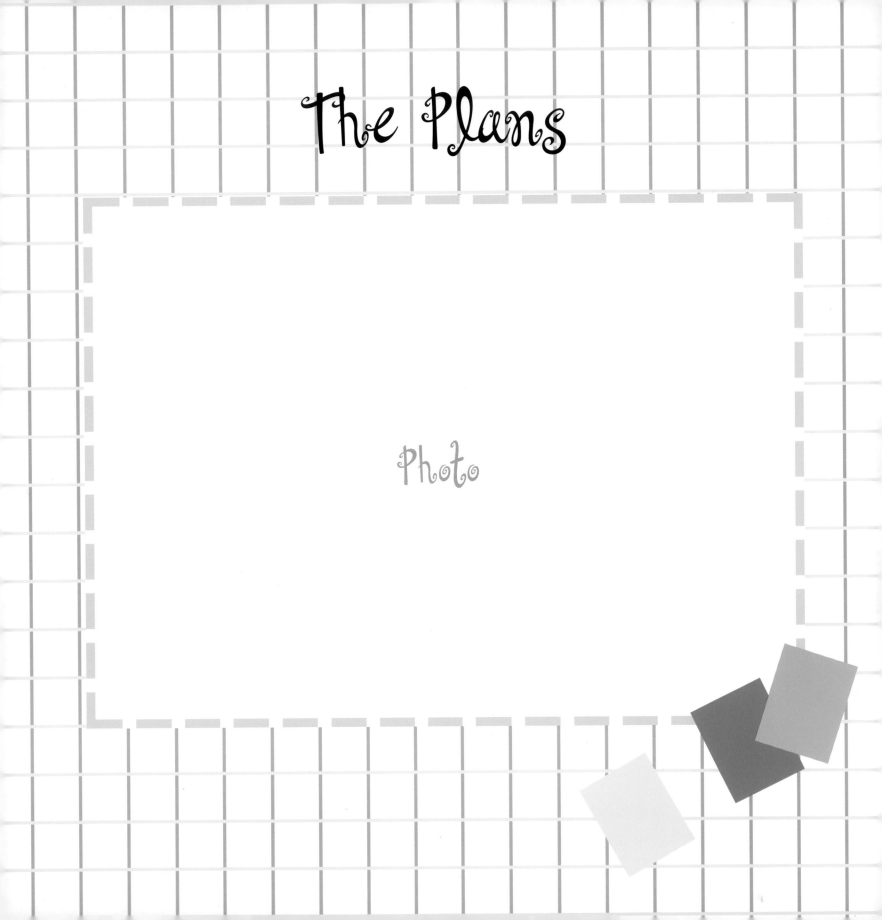

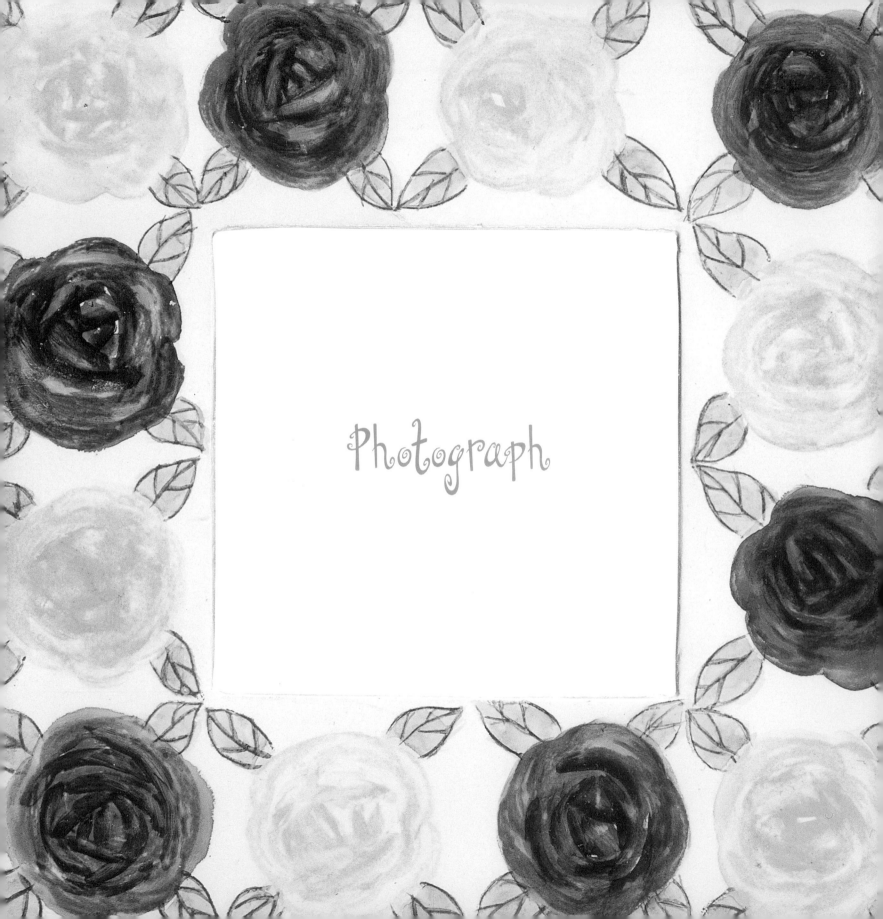

Photograph

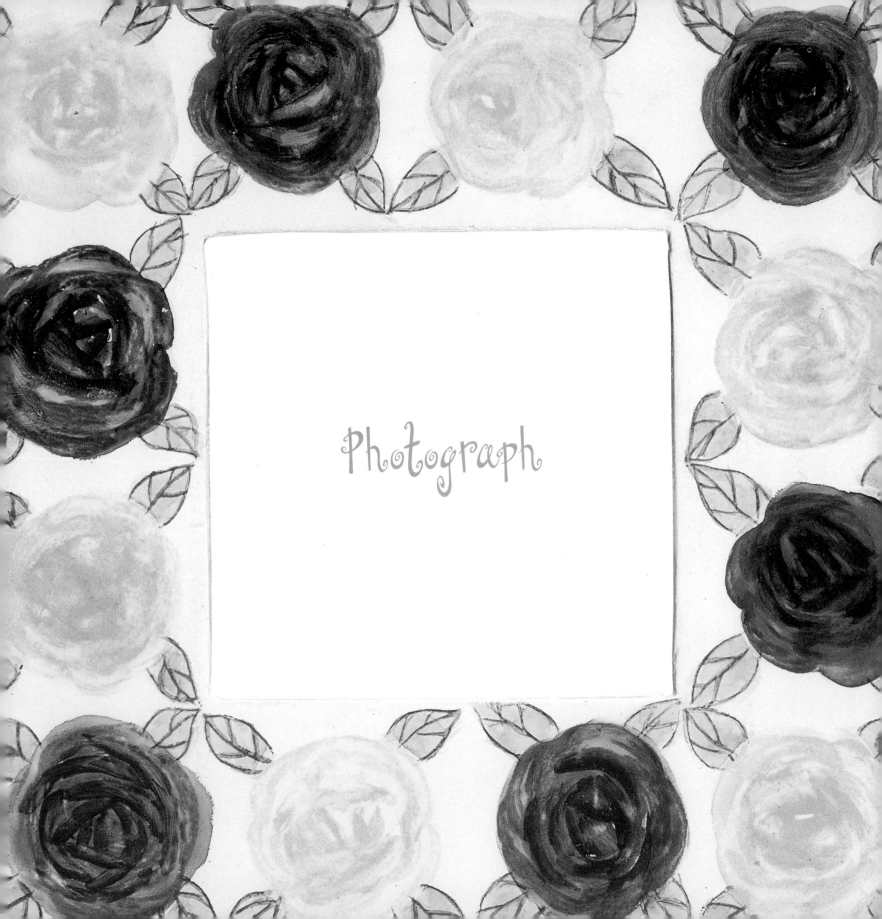

Photograph

My Thoughts and Feelings

at 6 months

_____

_____

_____

_____

_____

_____

_____

So What's in a Name?

Our favorite name

The history behind your name

Boys' Names

Girls' Names

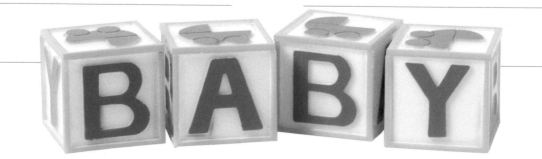

AUDREY • DOUGLAS • JASON • TYLER • DREW • MALORIE • JILLIAN • JACK • RACHEL • BRAD • ROBBIE • JOSIE • FRANK • SUE

HOLLIE • JASON • KARLIE • SUE • ROBERT • ELEN • MATHEW • PETE • ANNMARIE • KATHY • DEBORAH • DOUG • KAREN • BOB

JACKIE • EVA • TREVOR • MINDY • RYAN • ELIZABETH • HAILEY • ELENA • CARL • ROSEANNE • JUAN • FRANK • DEREK • ERICKA • ALEX

Ideas on Parenting

Mom

_____

_____

_____

_____

Dad

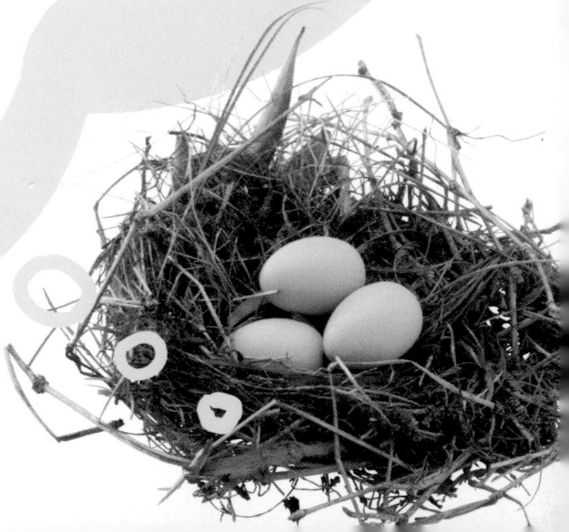

_____

_____

_____

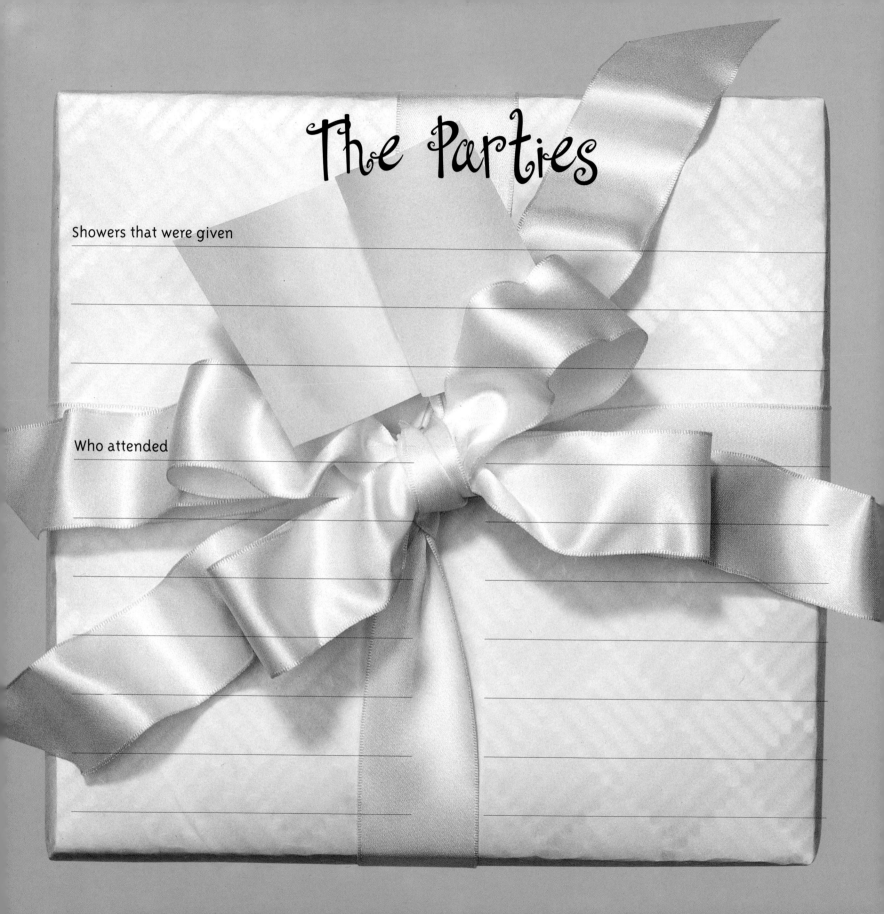

The Parties

Showers that were given
_____
_____
_____

Who attended
_____
_____
_____
_____
_____

The Invitation

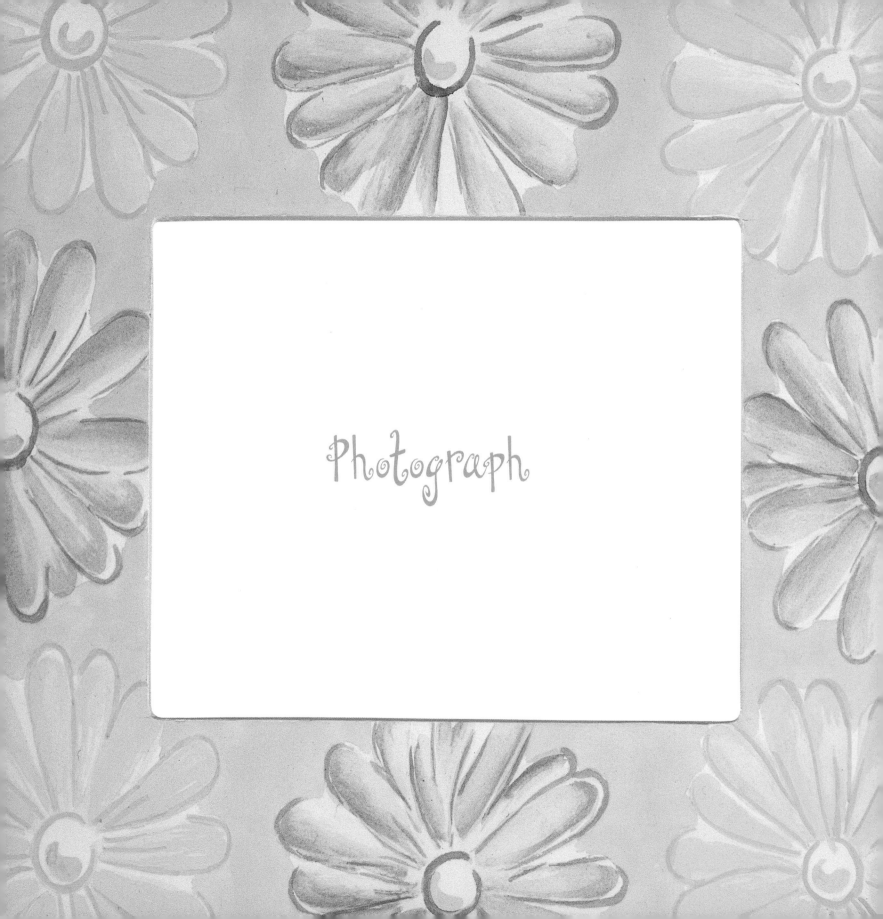

Photograph

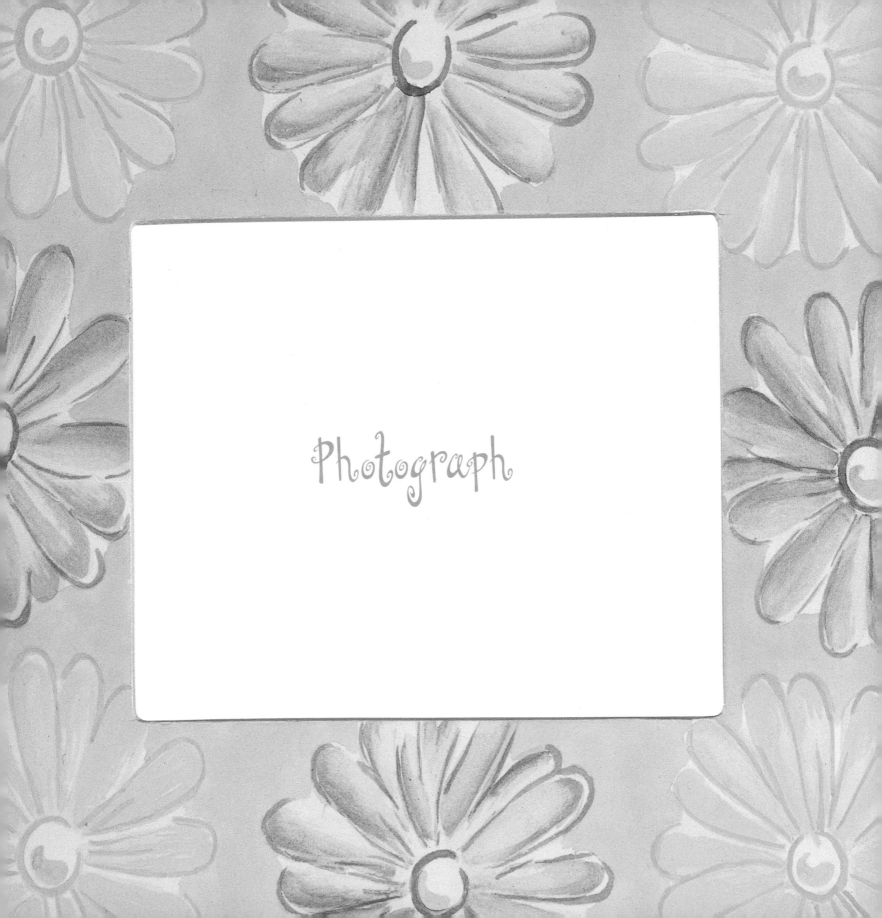

Photograph

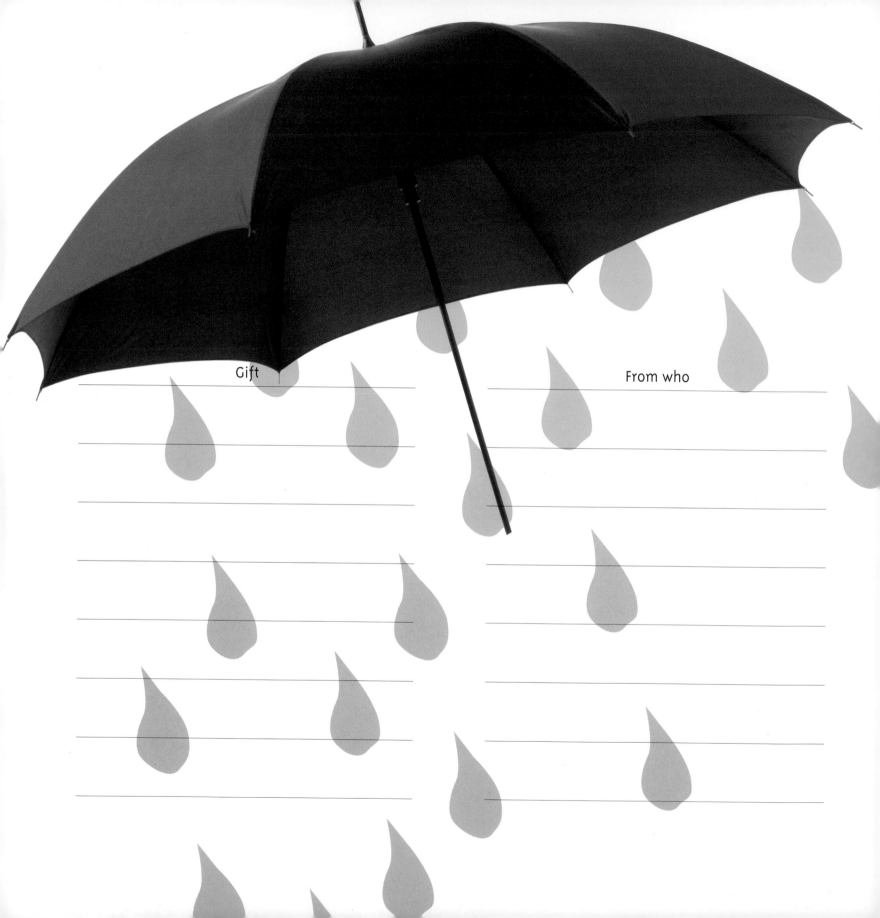

Gift

From who

Showering You With Gifts

Gift

From who

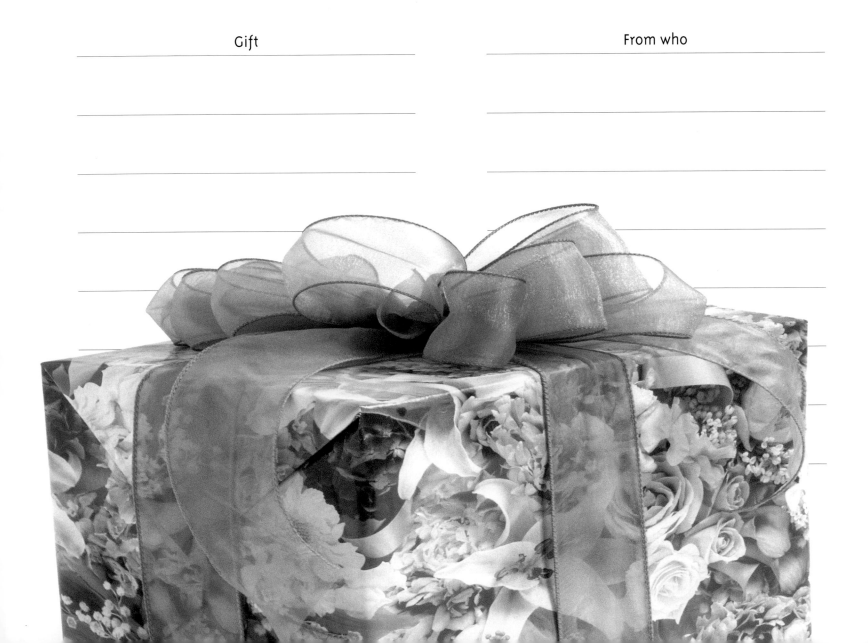

All in the Bag

Packing list for the big day

Who to Call for the Big Event

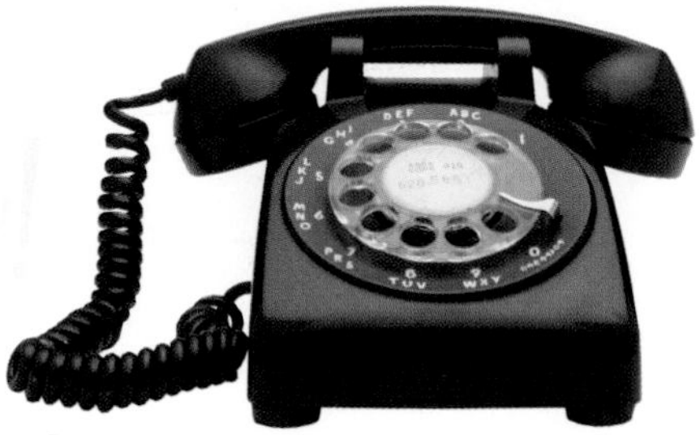

Name

Phone
_____

Name

Phone
_____

Name

Phone
_____

Name

Phone
_____

Name

Phone
_____

Name

Phone
_____

Name

Phone
_____

Learning to Breathe!

Classes I attended
_____

_____

_____

_____

_____

Coach
_____

_____

_____

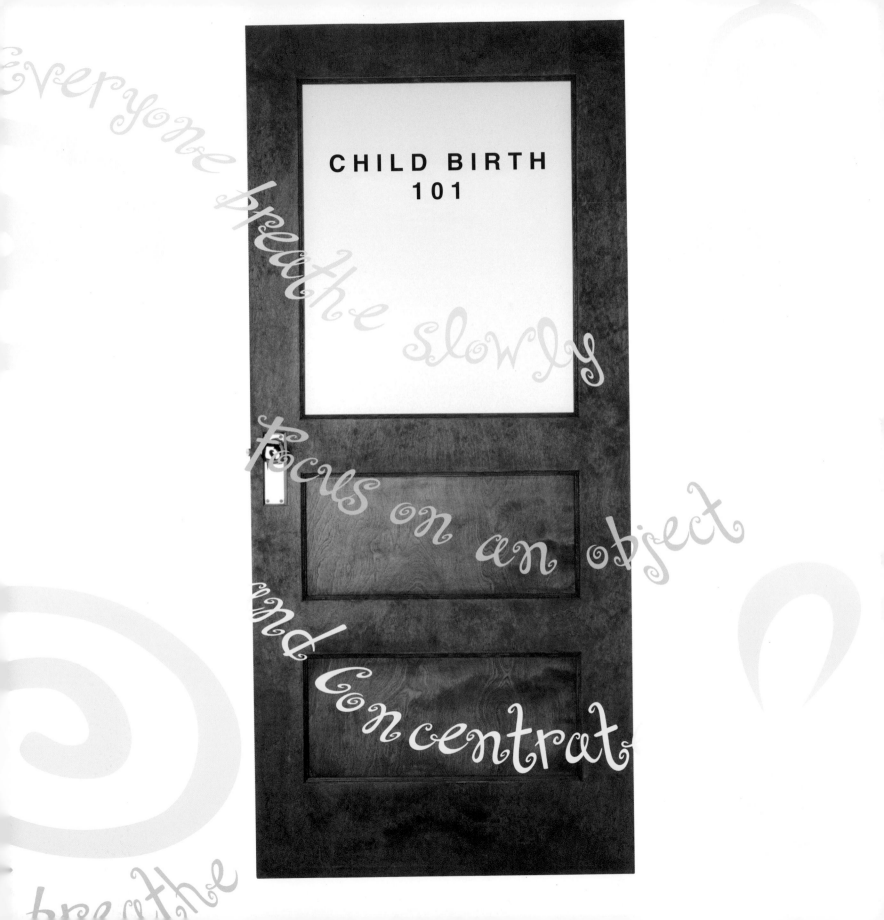

Photograph

Photograph

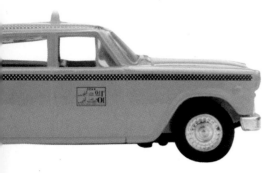

It's Time!

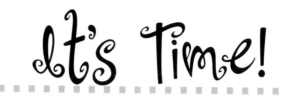

When it happened
_____

Where I was
_____

How I got to the hospital or birth center
_____

How long to get to the hospital or birth center
_____

How far apart my contractions were when we left
_____

Doctor
_____

What helped me most during labor
_____

_____

People who were there
_____

_____

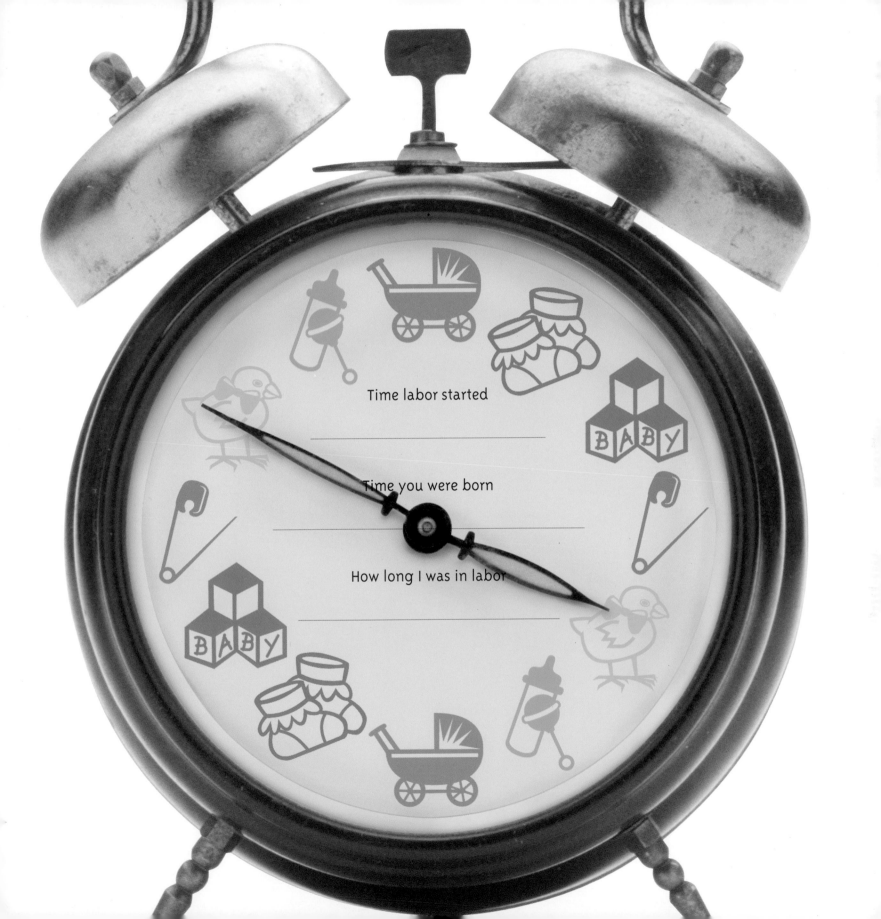

Time labor started

_____

Time you were born

_____

How long I was in labor

_____

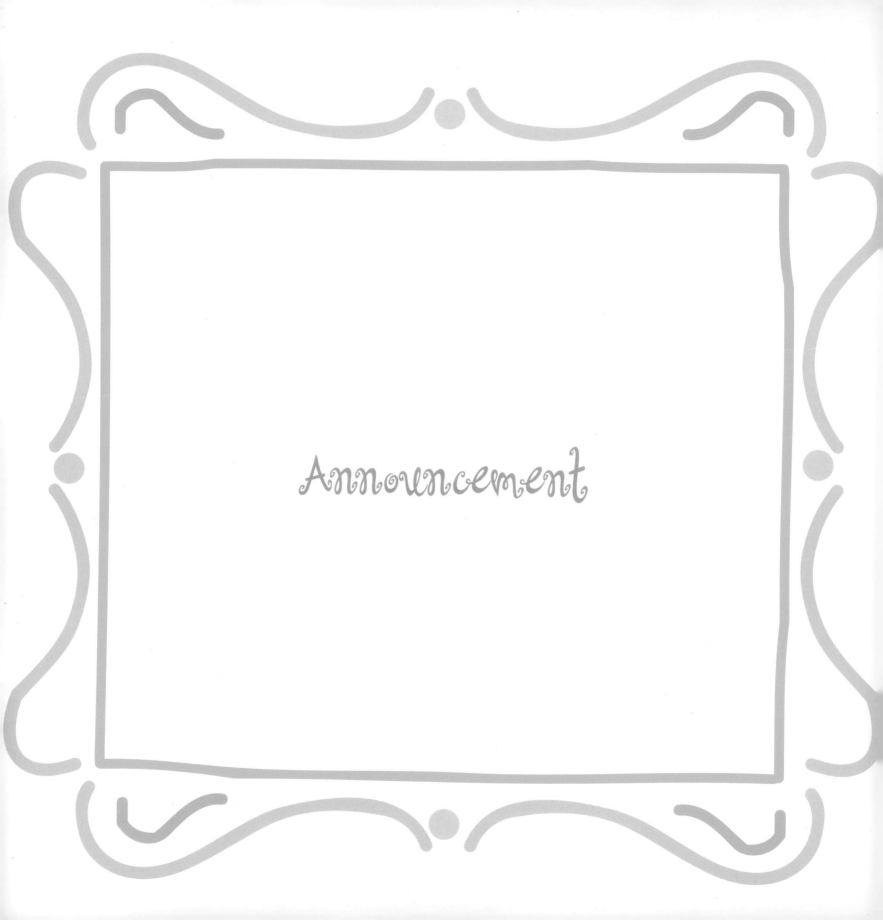

Announcement

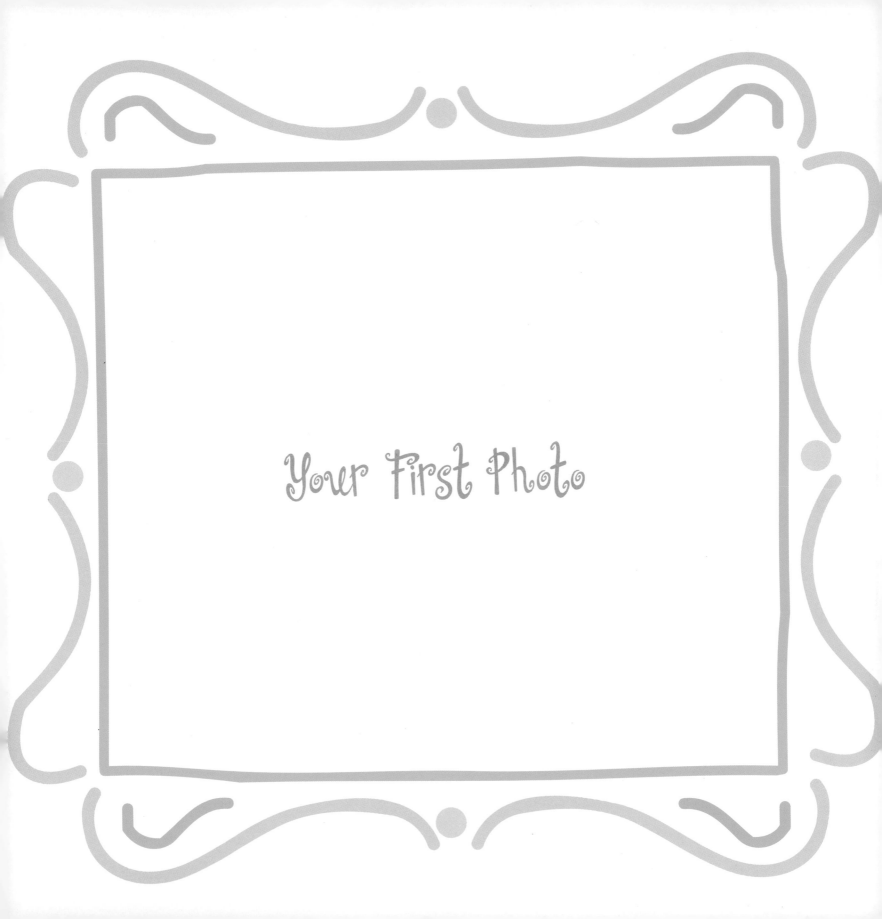

Your First Photo

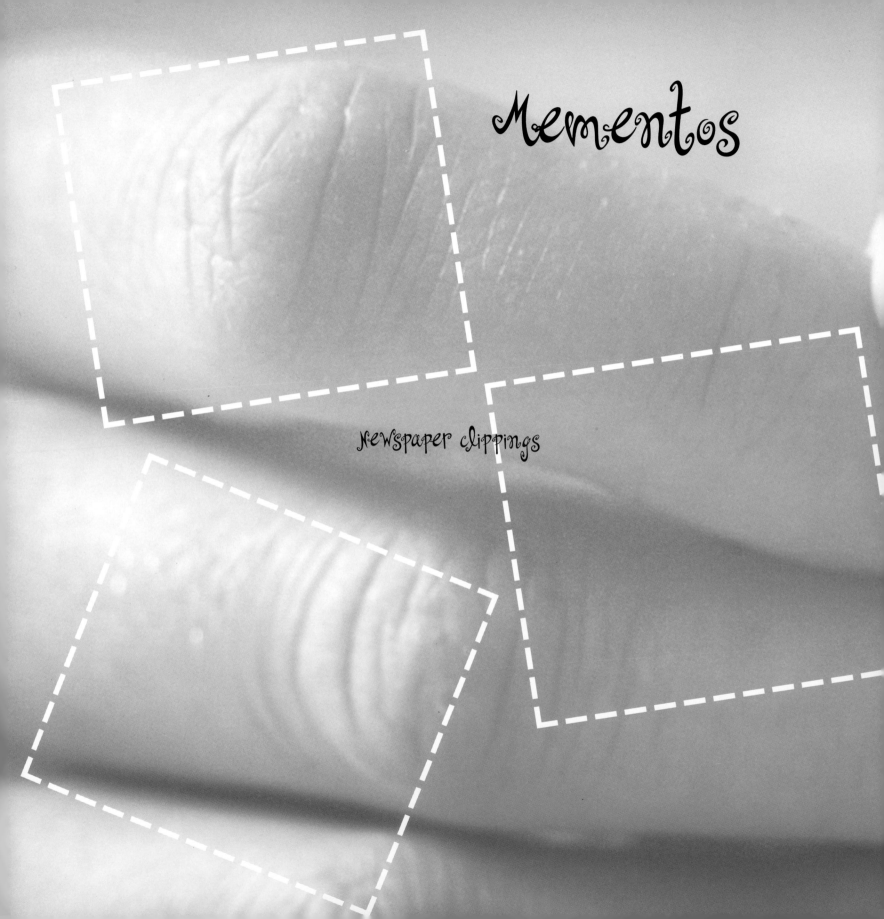

Mementos

Newspaper clippings

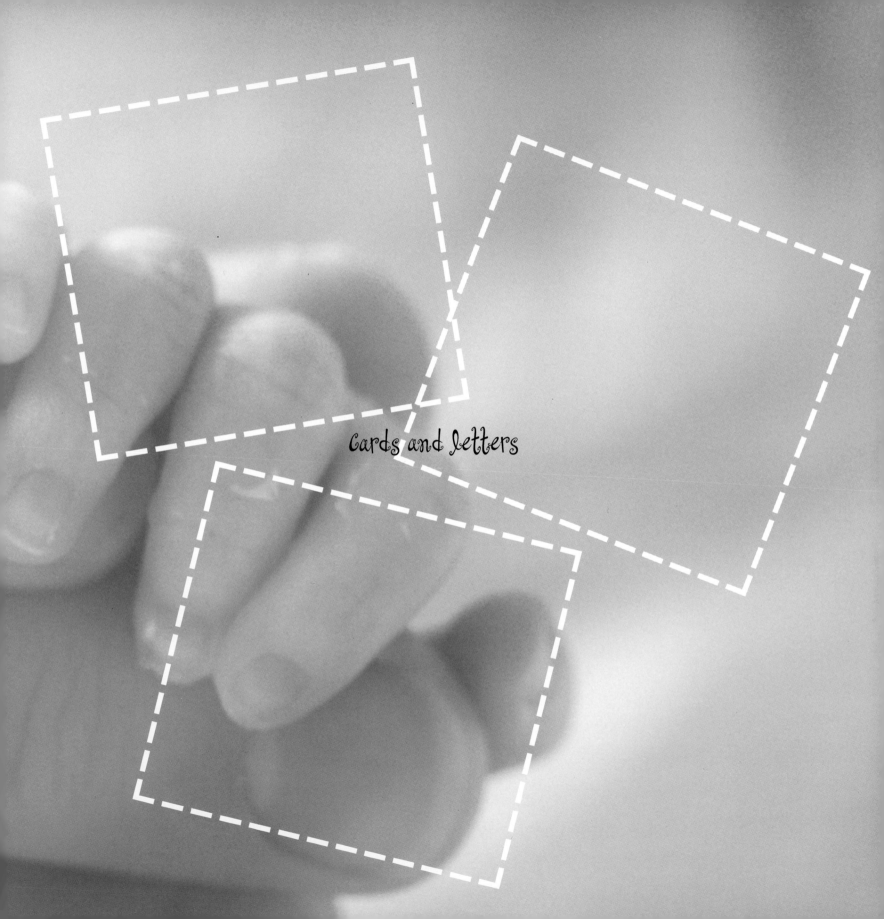

Cards and letters

Happy Birth Day to You

Your birth date

You weighed

Your birth time

You were this long

Other distinguishing features

As You Step Into The World

President

World leaders

National issues

International issues

Price of gasoline

Hit show

Big movie

Popular songs

Mood
_____

Energy
_____

Waist size/Weight gain
_____

Notes
_____

_____

Mood
_____

Energy
_____

Waist size/Weight gain
_____

Notes
_____

Month by Month

Mood
_____

Energy
_____

Waist size/Weight gain
_____

Notes
_____

_____

Mood
_____

Energy
_____

Waist size/Weight gain
_____

Notes
_____

_____

Mood _____

Energy _____

Waist size/Weight gain
_____

Notes _____

_____

3

Mood _____

Energy _____

Waist size/Weight gain
_____

Notes _____

_____

4

Mood _____

Energy _____

Waist size/Weight gain
_____

Notes _____

_____

5

Mood _____

Energy _____

Waist size/Weight gain
_____

Notes _____

_____

6

Mood _____

Energy _____

Waist size/Weight gain
_____

Notes _____

_____

4

Mood _____

Energy _____

Baby weight _____

Notes _____

Post Partum

Available Record Books from Havoc

Animal Antics-Cat
Animal Antics-Dog
Couples
Girlfriends
Golf
Grandmother
Mom
Mothers & Daughters
My Pregnancy
Our Honeymoon
Retirement
Sisters
Teacher
Traveling Adventures
Tying The Knot

HAVOC PUBLISHING
9808 Waples Street,
San Diego, CA 92121